BE YOUR OWN ANGEL is filled with wisdom and insight, and...[will] help women find the faith and courage to make the journey.

—George B. Friend, M.D., F.A.C.S.,
St Joseph's Medical Center, South Bend, Indiana

I awoke from my first cancer surgery to find my hospital room walls plastered with Nancy Swan Drew drawings delivered by Nancy to my husband to cheer me up and remind me that "tough cookies never crumble." This book will give to the world what she gave to me.

—Mary Jo Halbritter, *6-year cancer survivor*

It's very hard to wade through the fear and sadness and anger, but this little book gives hope as women with breast cancer see themselves on every page and realize they are not alone. Every single page is full of great wisdom...what a gift!

—Jennifer Donner, *caregiver*

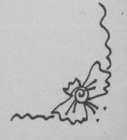

BE
YOUR
OWN
ANGEL...

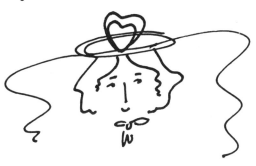

Snippets for
tough cookies
(Breast Cancer Soldiers)

by NANCY SWAN DREW

Celestial ARTs
Berkeley/Toronto

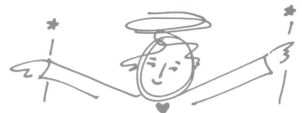

Celestial Arts
P.O. Box 7123
Berkeley, CA 94707
Library of Congress Cataloging
in Publication Data on file with
the publisher.
A HEART + STAR Book
First printing, 2000
Printed in Hong Kong
1 2 3 4 5 6 7 - 04 03 02 01 00

THis
little Book
is dedicAted And
Belongs
to

- - - - - - - - - - -

Feel veRy FRee to coloR
these pAges with the
indestnuctible enengy
youR liFe possesses.

youR FRiend,
Nancy S. Drew
x o x o x

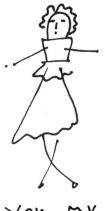

you, my
precious new
friend, are a

GEM

*

to keep forever
and always.

★ 🐌 ★

Introduction

Every woman lives a life...
worrying ✿
a little bit or a lot about
WHAT IF?

Through my art I have met
many remarkable women,
young and more seasoned,
who have faced breast
cancer with dignity and
a reservoir of enormous
strength... A true wonder-
ment to me, until now!.! ✶
After an early detection, I'm
on my way to discovering
their secrets... Let me share
some of them with you,
dolly!
xox

The most important
battles in life Are
About "things" one can-
not see or touch...
"things" of the spirit
help you deal with
physical ROadblocks,
And when All is said
And done, these battles
will be won by youR
oh-so-victorious
Spirit !!

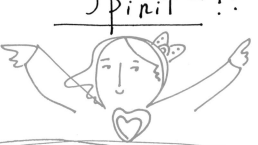

Believe, daRlin... believe.

FEAR would love
to keep you
company ... All day
And especially, darlin,
All Night. Please
refuse the invitation
And politely explain
that you Are too
busy keeping company
with
LiFe,
A wonderfully gracious
Guest you long to know
better.

Aunt Pearl* says...
"THERE'S
ALWAYS SOMEthing to
BAttle!!"

FOR NOW, dolly, this is
YOUR "something" AND, KNOWING
the CHAMP you ARE,
wINNING
is
A
SuRe thing!!

BRAVO

*
AuNt PeARl is A sweet
clone OF All those you've KNOWN
who ARe wiseR thAN the MAN iN
the MOON.

4

This is A time when
it's Really OK to
put your sweet self
FIRST.

If you ARe A mom,
this may be A very
Foreign exercise...
keep wor_king_ At it, doll.
For A little while it's

_____'s world.
YOUR NAme

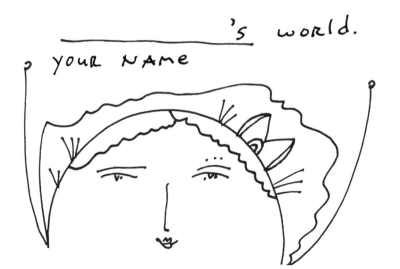

5

If you're having one of "those" days... go ahead, have a big piece of three-layered chocolate cake. It doesn't have to be your Birthday to celebrate!! No Sir!

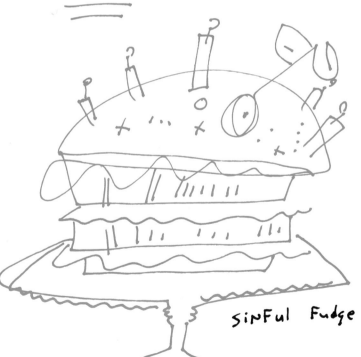

SinFul Fudge

Consider the MANY,
MANY contributing FActorS
to this Chapter:
genetics, environment,
some personal choices,
And the
BRoAd
mystery of Life itself.
THiS is NoT youR
FAuLt.
No, it isn't, darlin!

This unexpected journey
will give you A New
WARdRobe oF cRystAl-cleAR
Spectacles
to see the world ANew,
FRESH,
ANd Lovingly Yours!!

8

We All go through lAyers
oF ANger ANd SAdNesS...
the SooNeR you peel them
AwAy... the SooNeR you will

be FREE !!

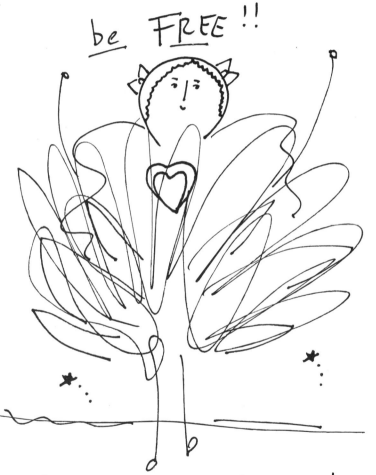

ONLy you, sweet ANgel,
CAN decide wHeN ANd How.

Before B.C. (breast cancer) there were good days and not so good. This practical mix carries on, dolly. You've dealt with it before and you surely will now.

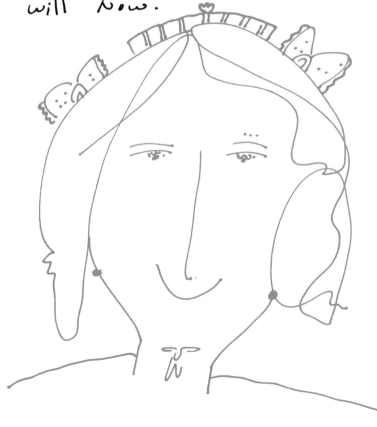

Faith
is believing that David
did defeat his Huge
FOE...
And you, darlin,
will, too.

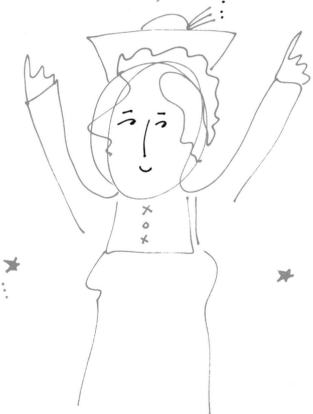

Your Recent News
is
<u>Not</u>
A Farewell Notice!
NO MA'AM,

No Missy...
only A zig And zag in
your life's tour de force.

detour

Rethink disappointment,
Anger, and Resentment
in
your
life...

Imagine these feelings
in a hot air balloon
Rising to the skies as
you stand atop an
emerald green hill,
basking in a sunshine
you've never known...
Nice !!!

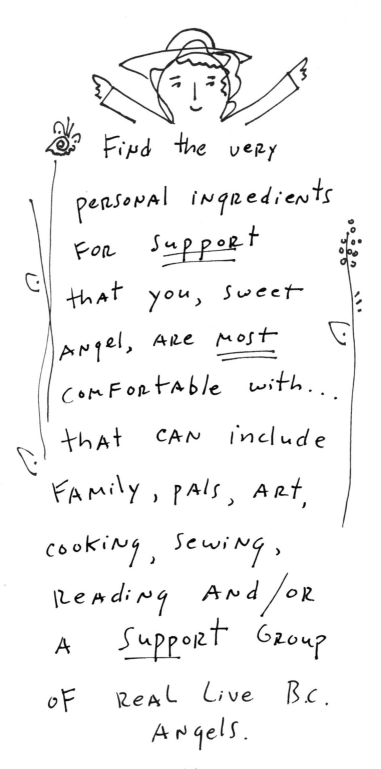

Find the very
personal ingredients
for Support
that you, sweet
Angel, are most
comfortable with...
that can include
Family, pals, art,
cooking, sewing,
reading and/or
a Support Group
of real Live B.C.
Angels.

True peace
runs deep
inside of you.
Find it,
dolly.

excavate diligently

This is A ducky time
to send hAnd-penned
pRoclAMAtions of love
to those who MAtteR.
Of counse, they MAy
already know how you
feel About them ... Still
A love letter is A
Beautiful
GIFt.

Dear susAn,
you are So very
important to
Me! I love
you big time!

Remember that when Family members try to Rise to the occasion... And make life perfect... Old Habits do Not vanish over-night. Forgive them when they stumble And know that PERFECT is only A word in the dictionary.

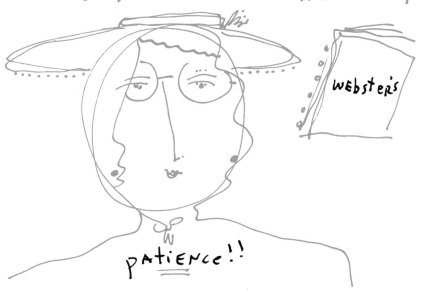

WEBSTER's

PATIENCE!!

Reconnect with people
you've been missing. Time
and bizee living can
sometimes temporarily
derail an ongoing
conversation. Write
notes or letters on
beautiful papers and
MAIL!

paris

usa

18

Some of those you
MAY encounter might be
unsure of how to handle
your news... let your
best "CAN·DO" attitude
prevail... even if theirs
slips a bit.

★

OH deAR...
how ARE you
doing?
MMM...
I've
heARd,
well,
you
know.

PREtty
well!!
thank
you!

SOME FOLKS let their own
FEARS CONFUSE them a bit.

15

Trust your very
own instincts...
take notes, ask
questions... All of
them. Sift through
And talk about
your Feelings!!
Pick people to listen
who do not Need hearing
Aids.

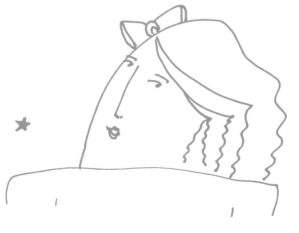

Develop A Mental
REFLex 🌀 that Rejects
All horror stories
or BAD NEWS hAnded to
you by well-meaning
folks. You ARE different
And will be just
Fine,
dolly... just Fine!

Your sailboat sails like
no other.

Make TEATIME A part of EACH day... it will calm And soothe!
Take a spot of REspite, dArlin !!

Feel AS Free AS A
Butterfly

to SAY NO... SAVE your
energy for whAt you
Need
And
Desire!

WhoA !! SORRy... NO CAN do,
Not this time... perhAps
Next time!

THis is youR
TiMe iN LiFe
to
BENd
like A seASONed
WiLLoW
TRee!

Ready... sET...   Go, dolly!!

xox

How deep is your
well of ANGER, dolly?
CRANK, ANd pull, ANd
empty...

Bucket
by
Bucket !!

THen ...

ReFill this Well with
wonder.

SURGERY...

Not NECESSARily youR IDEA OF A Respite FRom zooming + Zipping Routines, but oH so uAluAble FoR those MANy glorious HolidAys... strAight AheAd.!!

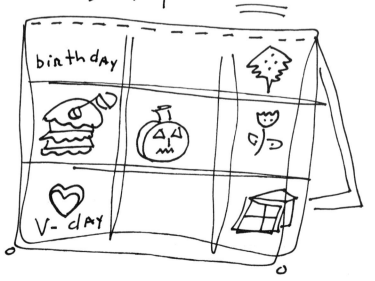

birthdAy

V-dAy

A hospital visit promises
you ROOM SERVICE,
darlin . . .
Room Service!!
Relax and push those
CALL
Buttons...

RELY ON OTHERS.

Trust your Doctors
And nurses... They
wear invisible medals
of honor As they
lead your ARMY
toward Victory!!!

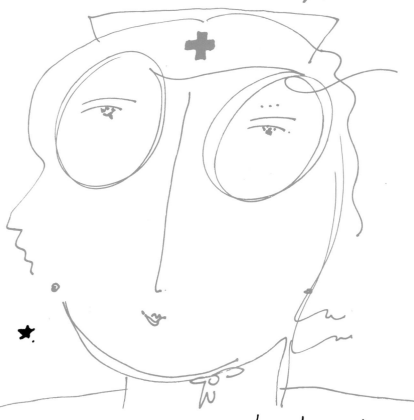

And of course, dArlin, Always
trust yourself, First.

Every individual is a
unique case. Statistics are
measurements a little
like dress sizes...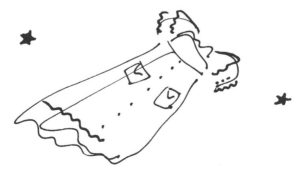
Approximate, variable, and
largely dependendent upon the
tailoring and fabric for
      Best
      Results...

Design your own ward-
Robe of Hope, and
wear it well !!!

Delivered Floral Arrangemen[t] give those FTD Ads on TV a new power.

MANY... MANY people Love you!!

FOR YOU

P.S. If you feel up to it, call the florist and compliment them on their artistry!!

While waiting for TEST RESULTS... Remember this... A zillion years from now, when you are residing in a real Honest - to - goodness PARAdise...

your TIMEX will be happily still.

Hush...
And do not worry.

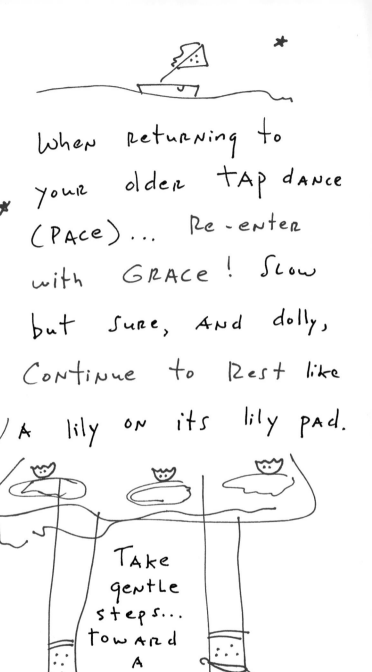

When returning to your older tap dance (pace)... Re-enter with GRACE! Slow but sure, and dolly, Continue to Rest like a lily on its lily pad.

Take gentle steps... toward a New normalcy.

Rest when you must...
PLAY AND RUN AS you
CAN... TREAT yourself
A little each day like
A kid ON CHRISTMAS
MORNing...

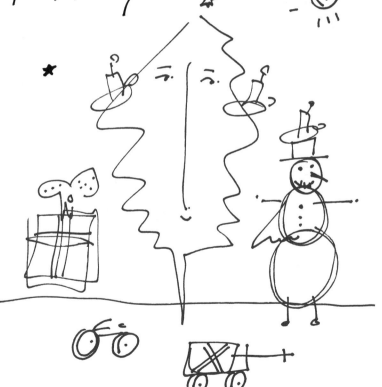

Every day you rise And
shine, light An invisible
cANdle deep inside your
spirit...

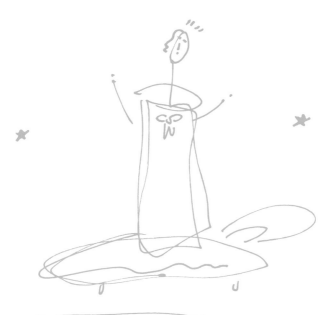

No MATTeR whAt cloudy ShAdows
loom NeARby, youR wAy
will be cleAR, dolly.

BELIEVE it, dolly!
CHEMO is A GiFt to
you... See it WRApped
up iN the pAges of
youR FutuRe, with
A SAtiN bow oF well-
Ness ANd HiGH, High
pRomise!!

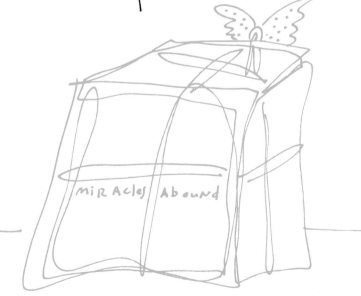

miR Acles AbouNd

Invisible gifts Abound
And your Courageous
heart will — day by
day — MAke them
visible And ReAL !!

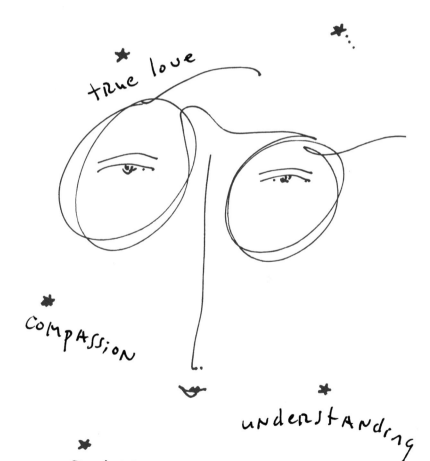

true love

compassion

understanding

peAce

you MAy hear of A zillion
possible Side effects
ReIAted to tReAtments...

Take this INFo with A
gigANtic gRAiN oF
SAIt.

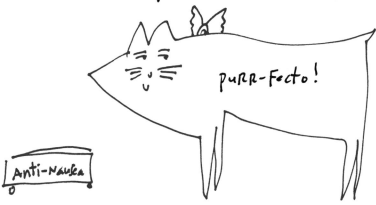

MODeRN medicine is
Full oF New, gReAt
strategies to MiNiMize
these "possibilities ..."

puRR-Fecto!

Anti-NAusea

Right this very minute, brilliant, hardworking people are doing Research to Find better Treatments and a cure for Breast Cancer. 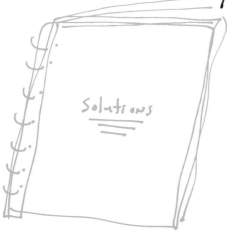   Very soon, things will be better for one and all. THANK goodness!

Solutions

PLAN ahead FOR youR days OF tReAtMent: tidy up youR Nest... do groceRy shopping... And most importAnt, sit down with youR sweet selF And ReAdy youR mind, body, And heArt foR this mission - possible towaRds wellNess.

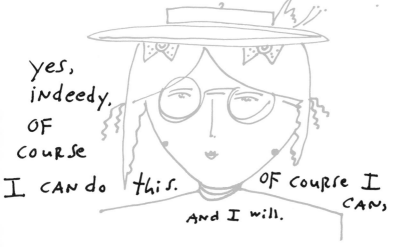

yes, indeedy. OF couRse I cAN do this.

OF couRse I cAN,

And I will.

IVs during treatments...

IF it is A task for the nurse to find A good entry vein... Suggest A hot pad or request A veteran nurse who is AN expert At this... there is one... so speak up, dolly (no one likes to be poked, really!) xox

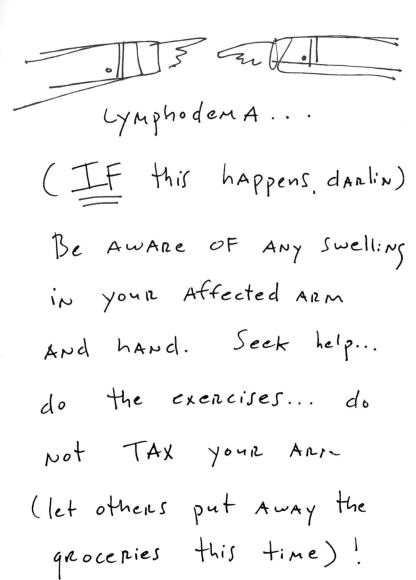

LymphodemA . . .

(IF this happens, darlin)

Be AWARE OF ANY swelling
in your Affected ARM
And hand. Seek help...
do the exercises... do
not TAX your Arm
(let others put Away the
groceries this time)!
Like other circumstances
in life... Find A FoRMulA
FoR MANAGEMENT!
xox

RELAXATION...

is A Lost ARt that CAN be LEARNed.
Let this be A Big PARt OF your dAiLy
HOMEWORK !!

breathe in 1·2·3
slowly...
breathe out 1·2·3

Repeat

Fighting FAtigue * is your New pARt-time job. Like All things worth doing, it will require An extrA Push...

And women, dolly, Are experts At this...

Experts!!

Solitude
is simply being Alone
with a very best
Friend...

Yourself!!!
Enjoy it, darlin...

44

Soapy Soap operas
can make dark days
look like a day at
the beach... Such
naughty stories in
lovely settings are
truly high fictional
Art.

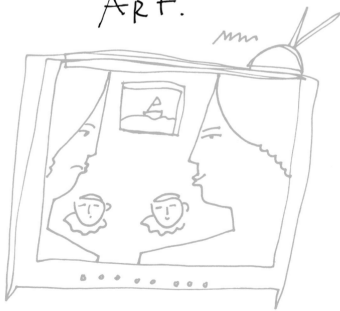

Uh-oh... DAytime
TELevision MAy
become youR best
FRiend... be glAd it's
oNly temporARy!
ChANNel suRf foR
the good stuff, dolly!

*

HGTV

PBS

Movie CLASSics

it's
out
there!!

MOVIES
ARE MINI-VACATIONS...
Select good ones!!!
READ Reviews carefully!
Bring Fruit AND WATER
to keep you in fine
COMPANY...
Although popcorn NEVER
ever FAils!

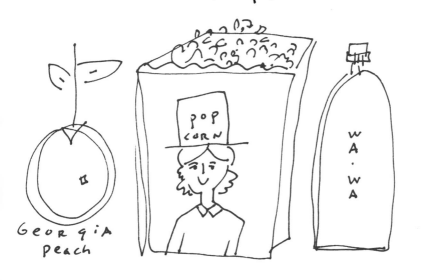

GEORGIA
peach

POP CORN

W A . W A

Look Around your Abode...

Putter And Purge...
redecorate ... shop A
little bit... Doll up your
life with nice changes
that bring A quiet
BEAUTY
to your LAndscape...
inside
And
out!!

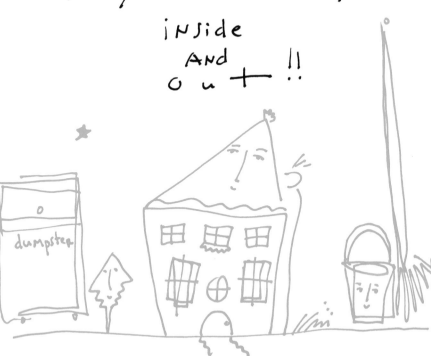

dumpster

During And
After your treatment,
begin A long-term vitamin
And nutrition plan to
support your Goood
Health.

GOALS
_____
_____
_____
_____
_____
_____
_____
_____

Begin... even IF slowly... begin.

Aunt Pearl says...
kiss the ticky-tacky
drive-thru goodbye and
embrace the produce
at your corner grocery!
Discover the magic of
HERbs...

Harvest only the best,
darlin!!

chives

thyme

basil

dill

cilantro

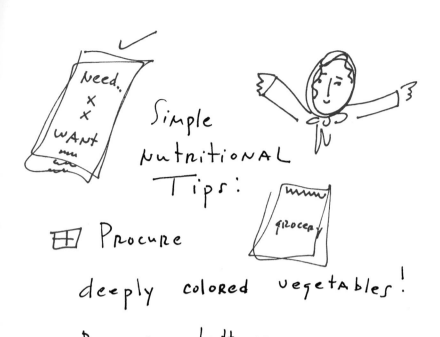

Simple Nutritional Tips:

⊞ Procure

deeply colored vegetables!

- Romaine lettuce
- Tomatoes
- spinach

⊞ Remember garlic and all fruits (Think Garden of Eve).

⊞ Treat yourself to the ORGANICALLY grown section!

BALANCE is your new culinary Trick!

DRINK WATER IN NIAGARA
FALLS FASHION... BE YOUR
VERY OWN CULLIGAN GAL!!.

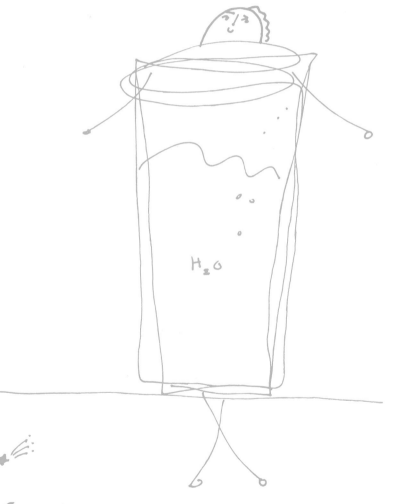

H_2O

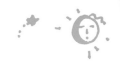

Darlin, Avoid a heavy
diet of CNN and other
News broadcasts...
especially before
Bed time!!

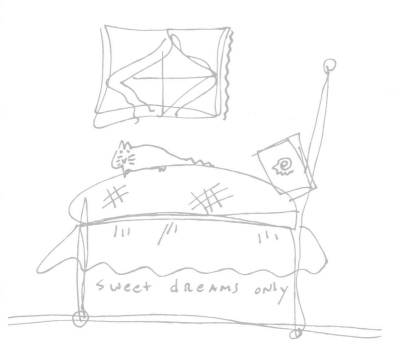

sweet dreams only

IN the middle of the Night... iF you find your MIN̲d̲ dANcing the two-step with FEAR itself... S̲E̲E̲ yourself on the other side of this contest * swing dAncing with HOPE... well And hAPPy AgAiN.

ALL beHer!! Now!

FiNiS

PRAYER is conversation
with A higher power
who sits FAIR And
Square in the driver's
Seat... CARRY on A
loving dialogue And
know that your voice
is heard!!

Loud And Clear!!

You don't
Need to be
IN A cHURch
OR TEMple
to
chit·
cHAt.

Fact :

The Mind can only enter-
tain one guest-thought
at a time... Invite
only the very best in,
dolly!!

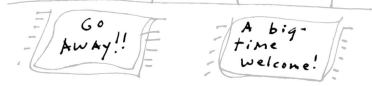

Negative
thoughts

positive
thoughts

Go
Away!!

A big-
time
welcome!

Do not let worry bankrupt your very dear and special savings account...

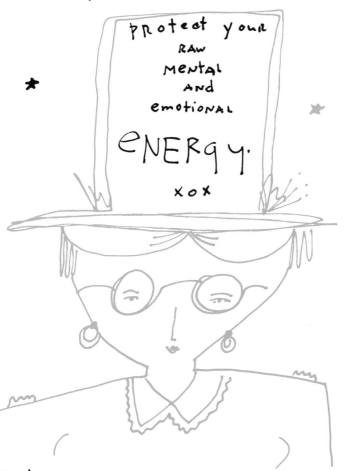

Protect your
RAW
MENTAL
AND
emotional
ENERGY.

xox

BALANCE FACT + FICTION with AN optimistic vision, doll.

Your imagination can take you anywhere, Darlin! Where would you like to go?!!

PERSONAL PASSPORT

I remember when I loved to go to the beach... And make a baker's dozen of Mud pies.

PLAN A Holiday For the
end oF your treatment...
it can be As tiny As A
trip to the beAch or As
grAnd As A tour oF

ＥＵＲＯＰＩＡ !
_____

MARK your cAlendAr...
And look forward to
A   celebration !!

Look !!

Practice, as **best** you can, keeping up your regular routine...
grocery shopping, errand running... Slowly but surely
life will return to better than
NORMAL!!

Rediscover
the Art of Grown-up
* Napping !!!

Zzzz...

...Zzz

zzz...

m m

meow-princess

There is no crystal
Ball !!

Remember this, and
let each day fly
high like a red, blue,
and golden kite against
Dairy Queen clouds...
Hurry, doll... and bring
plenty of String !!!

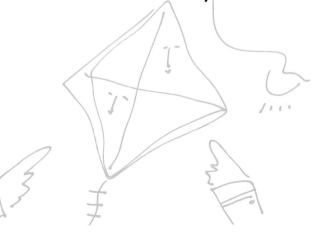

When you look in the
          MiRROR,
Remember this, dARLin...
You ARe A beautiful
Spirit   iN A ReNted body,
which is temporARily undeR
          RenovAtioN...
Very vALuAble RehAb!!

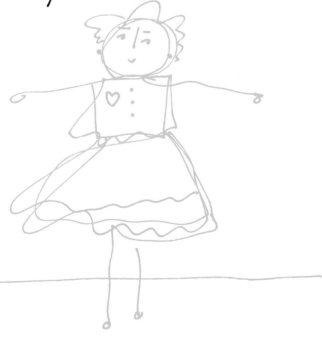

Laughing out loud
is A miraculour
nonprescription drug!!
So is letting your voice
Reach
the
tree tops
with
tornado
Force!

However you wish,

HAR...

HO·HO·HO...HARDY HAR

"BLAST OFF" those MANY PASSIONS
that seem unspeakable.

Believe it or NOT...
there is usually something
FUNNY
deep inside your own
PERSONAL serving of
LiFe's
Bittersweet Porridge.

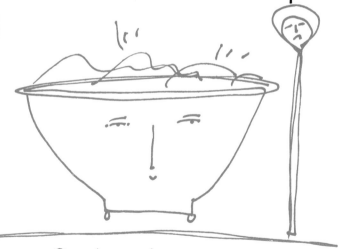

Look,
dARLiN...
it's there, I promise.

Pamper your Pearly
whites... Brush Full-
time throughout the
day
And smile,
darlin... smile!!!

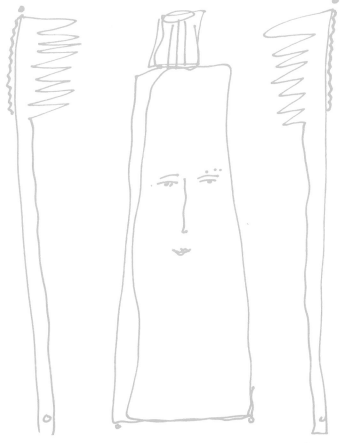

share that lovely spirit!

MAKeup

CAN peRK A gAl up!!
PLAy with it As you
oNce did At youR
moTheR's vAnity.

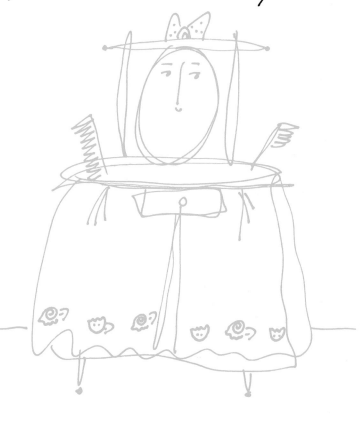

MINOR FACtoids...

* dry skin may visit...
baby yourself with creamy
creams!

* As your hair departs,
there may be some itching
And New sensations.
Once again, call out your
creamery!

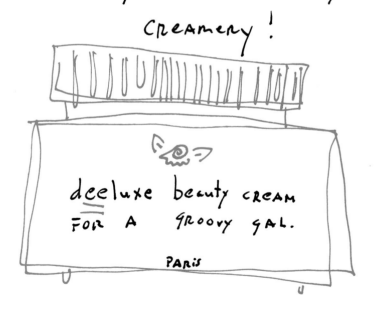

deeluxe beauty cream
FOR A groovy gal.

PARiS

No woman in her right mind misses shaving her legs.

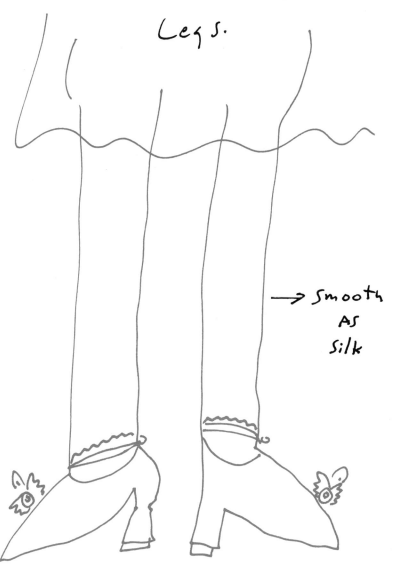

→ Smooth as silk

Stay in your right mind, darlin... it suits you.

69

If your hairdo is
temporarily on vacation,
discover scarves... hats...
perhaps MADONNA - or
TINA TURNER - like wigs.
Play dress up FOR REAL,
dolly !!

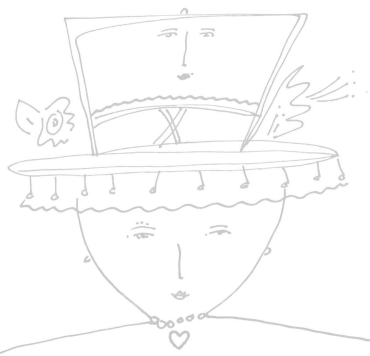

And take your very own
HEAD - dressing vacation !

If your treatment means a very short time without hair... consider cutting your hair or even shaving in "GI JANE" fashion. Demi Moore was one tough cookie ... As you are, dolly!! Easy on the eyes too! You are

BEAUTIFUL!!!

The day will come,
dolly, when your hair
will sprout like A
Georgia peach, And
your eyelashes will
curl up Bette Davis style,
And your step will
bounce once Again As
your perky self is
BORN
ANEW !!

DARLIN... YOUR HAIR will grow back in the blink OF AN EYE. IMAgine it blowing in the wind, As you watch YOUR CARES FLOAT up to the HeAvens.

Angst

Worry

guilt

Regret

Anger

FEAR

BAh-bye! So...long!!

Beauty is All About you... in ARt, music, buildings, And NAtuRe ... in the eyes oF those you love And even in the eyes oF StRAngeRs. Seek this divine beauty. Like An umbRellA oF NORtheRn stARs oN A cleAR Night... its poweR will pRotect And guide you, dolly.

Look up !!!!

You ARE Now EARNing A
New degree: Ph.D. in
TREASuRing."
nothing in life matters
unless it is treasured...
Moments, beauty,
people!! Discovering
what you value the
most on this earth is
well worth knowing...
DR. TREASuRe!!
BRAvo!

Radiation...

A quiet time each day to lie still, rest, and pretend you are at the beach where Sunscreen is of

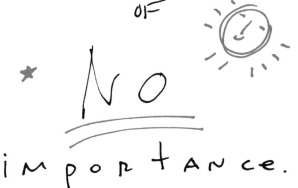

No

importance.

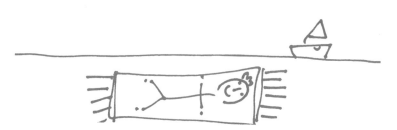

For Each And every
daily trip to RADiAtion
plan A little extrA trip just
For Fun on the wAy home.. shop
At A FARMER's MARket or your
fAvorite Antique spot, or get
A mAnicuRe, or have teA
with A pAl. PeRhaps just tAke
A new roAd home...
explore. Be A free butterfly. ...

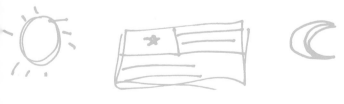

When listening to the
steady hum of the
Angel of Radiation,
imagine yourself in
a place you'd rather
be... that summer
cottage rental or
spring trip to the
shore. Let your
memory get very specific!
And Bingo .. you're done!

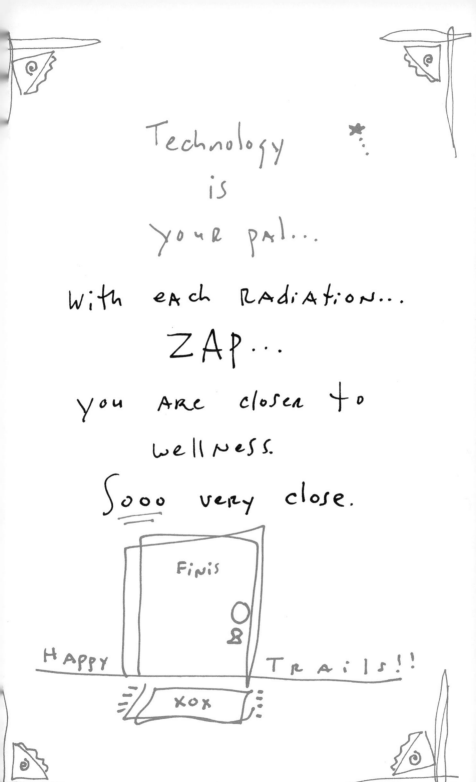

Technology
is
your pal...

With each RADIATION...
ZAP...
you Are closer to
wellness.

Sooo very close.

Finis

HAPPY   TRAils!!

XOX

RADIATION

CAN give you A New
devotion
And
Respect
FoR Skin Creams!!
And
Loverly
Lotions!

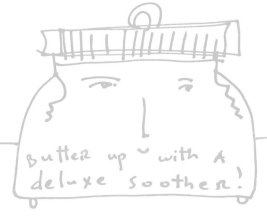

Butter up ~ with A
deluxe soother!

In the waiting room...
A beautiful woman said
that prescriptions nowadays
were so Expensive,
it would simply be

¢   Cheaper
                to
  ⫬   Die.   ⫬

¢   ¢   ¢
  "Just kidding!!!"

She said... gently.
    "Just kidding!"

A plus for RADIATION
patients is that if
you start READING A
LONG article or short
story in the lobby, you
CAN Always count on
finishing it the Next
dAy... or the Next... or
the one After that.

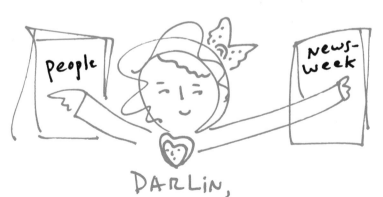

People

News-
week

DARLiN,
All good things take time.

Imagine

Hospital gowns as
a swishy DKNY
shift in a luxe silk-
and-linen blend...

Pearls
are optional,
dolly!!

oooo...   L.A., CA!

There should really
be a re-evaluation
of the music in
Doctors' offices... For
example, the tune
that's keeping my
anxious spirit company
right this minute is
"One Last Egg to Fry"...
WELL, I DON'T THINK
So, dolly! There are
a zillion more to scramble,
Flip, soufflé, and Quiche
Life up with! (Try yours
with a touch of Basil!)

Minimize Stress by Not
Owning
everyone else's mud puddle.

They, not you, are the
only ones who can dog-
paddle their way out.

★...

And now, more than ever,

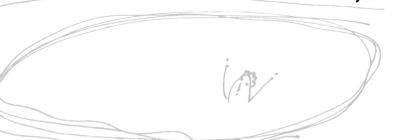

Let them become
Olympic swimmers, darlin'!

85

Dolly...
Which would you
prefer???
To BE HAPPY
OR
ALWAYS AND Absolutely
RiGHT ?

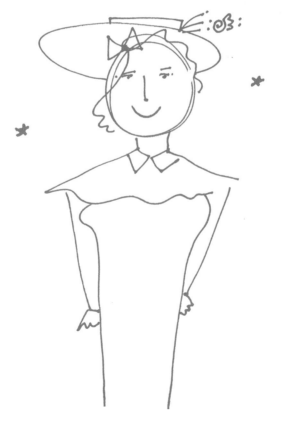

PL

Exercise in a glamorous
getup with a cute trainer
or take a nice walk
in blue jeans... You decide!
It's really all the same...
you know...
Motion, dolly...
Locomotion!!

Believe it or Not there
is joy in little projects
that have NAgged your
"To Do" ★
★ list...

cleaning A drAwer, going
through closets,
ORDeRing
the petite compARtments
of youR world so that
when you Really feel
better, you cAN go out
ANd PlAy!

xox

88

The trick to positive
thinking is to have
Huge Faith 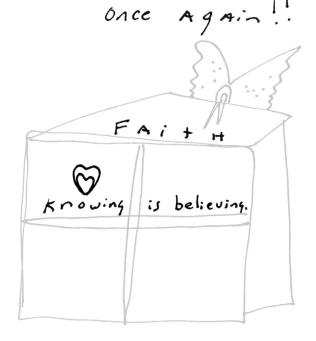 when days
are punk and gray...
BELIEVE that true happiness
will gift-wrap your
dreams
once again!!

FAITH

Knowing is believing.

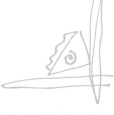

ALL
aboard...

Meow.

EMOTIONAL
TRAVEL
FActoid:

EVEN when things turn you
upside down... REMEMBER
that Right-side up is your
next stop.
whoa ... Hold on tight!!

90

THERE ARE NO VICTIMS,

ONLY
HEROES
AND
Sterling troopers!

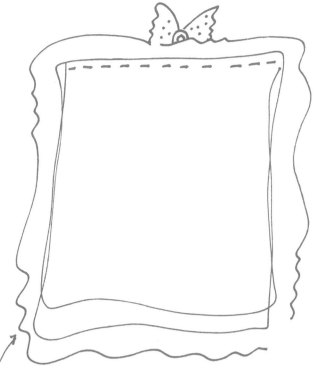

DRAW yourself or place photo Above!!

YOU ARE A TEACHER
NOW...
Showing the WAY along
this NEW PATH to All
who love you. Guide
them AS best you CAN
AS A MOM, sISTER, pAl,
daughteR, niece, OR Aunt!!
BRAVO, Ms. PRofessor
OF
CouRAge!!

P.S.
NOt All RoAds   ARe chosen.

NO
MATTER
How old you ARE todAy...
MotheR youR sweet SELF

★

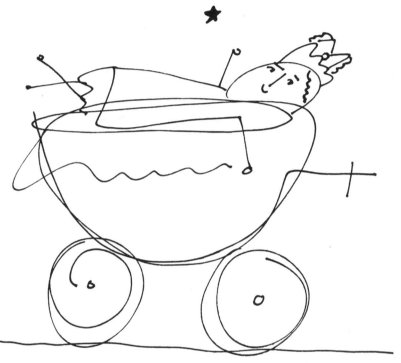

like you would A precious
NewboRN...
becAuse, dARliN... iN A wAy,
you ARe About to be
Reborn!!

FAST-FORWARD YOUR
HEART'S busy SOUL to
the end OF tREAtMent...

SOON,
dolly,
SOON
i̱t̲ will be ALL

FiNished!!

SEE!
you ARe
heRe, At the
beach
celebRAting.

Once your very, very
important treatments
cease... BEGIN AGAIN!
Baby your sweet self
into wellness... Run
Away on A petite
H O L i d A y
And
Rejoice!
You deserve it, yes
you do!!
Now go on, dolly, And
Have Big-time Fun!
It's out there just waiting
FOR your
company!

95

AFTER treatments, on to checkups!

B.C. Fall out

★

As time passes...

your life will, of course, be a different one. And it CAN

be a better life!!

Work like a pro

at Filtering the

worries and fears

that may cloud

your journey of

wide-awake Joy!

BREATHE deeply. ★ Relax

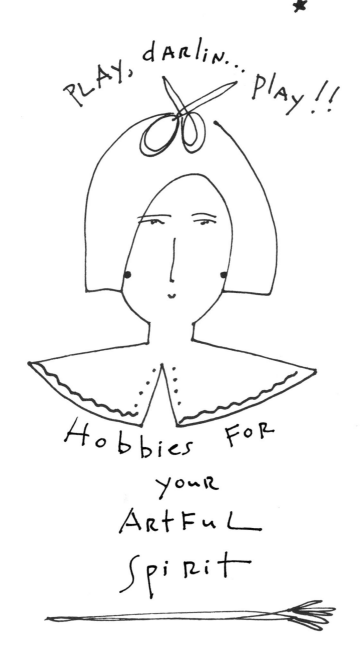

I. ✂

PLAY with ART
MATERIALS to MAKE
YOUR <u>OWN</u> thank-
you OR NOTE CARDS...
use collAge, old photos,
OR Simply dRAw ANd
coloR A MessAge oN
stuRdy PAPeRS...

photo-
copy OF
you As
A
child

I LOVE
YOUR ANGEL

H
E
A
R
T

CONSTRUC-
tion
PAPER
cut with
pinking
SheARS

II.

Decorate a box...
write your dreams and
hopes... even worries, and
store them there! Date
these secrets for future
reference, when all is
well again!   xox

→ buttons

→ Rick-
RACK

Susan's Better-

than-best thoughts

III.

Keep a record of all the things you want to do after you are well again... doll up a simple notebook with felt cut-outs... Picasso style! And script away!

TO-DO... SOON!

IV.

TAke All the gifts of
cheer, wisdom, And
hope And jot them
down on post-its!!
Post these on your
mirror, Fridge, kitchen
cupboard, back door,
And dashboard.
Wherever ! your eye
travels...

XoX

XoX

XoX

V.

Painting is very therapeutic! Paint ~~it~~ a chair, stool, box, lampshade, denim jacket, or stretched canvas! Become an artist of self-expression!

Lots of color!

use water-based paints!

VI.

CREAtive cooking!!
On those wonderful days
when you feel willing And
Able... open A favorite
cookbook or find A
New one! Explore the
ARtistry of blending
fine ingredients from
scratch, to make A
lovely dish...
Live, dARlin,
     Live!!

VII.

If you ever practiced sewing, knitting, needlepoint, cross-stitch, or crocheting, Now is the time to dive back in or LEARN A few basics!! Make something beautiful while your own beauty unfolds...

VIII.

Find a paint-your-own pottery studio in your neck of the forest. They are PURR-fect spots for your spirit to rest and create one-of-a-kind gifts for all those angels who love you so well. And remember to make an extra-special gift for your best angel, yourself, darlin'!

P.S. play like a little child where mistakes are invisible.

IX.

Decorate

A PROMISE JAR...
(ANy jAR will do)with
PAint, glue, etc... In
this FANcy vessel, write
little Notes OF promise
to yourselF... things
you will treAsure,
chAnge, ANd explore to
CHARM YOUR NEW
LiFe FORWARd
AS YOUR OWN true
ANqeL.
xox   xox

BE
yOuR
OWN
ANgeL...

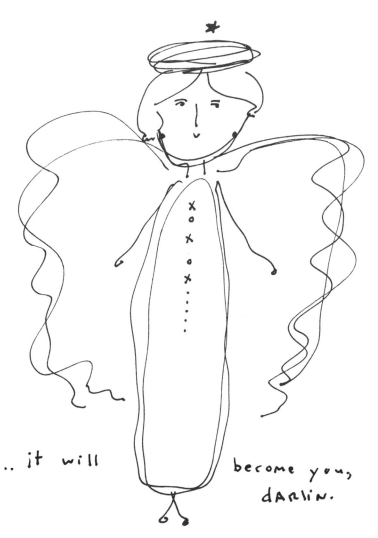

... it will become you, dARliN.

About the Author
And Artist... Nancy
Swan Drew is a
celebrated fine artist
and the author of The
Artful Spirit and First-
Aid kit for Mothers.
She has been practicing
being her own Angel
since the early detection
of Stage I Breast Cancer
in 1999. Prognosis is great...
(A trusty mammogram is
a loyal friend.) She gives
a bounty of love-pats
to all tough-cookie
soldiers whose spirits are
and always will be
Victorious! Bravo!

www.NancySwanDrew.com

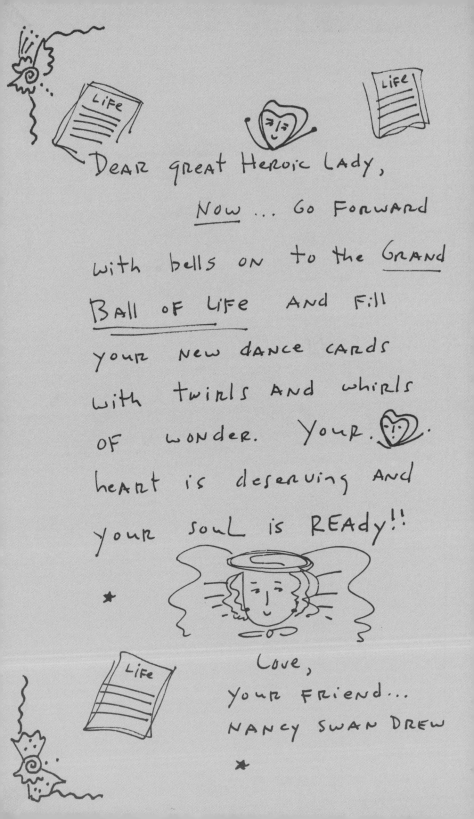

DEAR great HEROIC LADY,

Now ... GO FORWARD
with bells on to the GRAND
BALL OF LIFE AND Fill
your New dance cards
with twirls AND whirls
OF wonder. Your
heart is deserving AND
your souL is REAdy!!

*

Love,
your FRIEND...
NANCY SWAN DREW

*